Tales of the Exam Room Volume 1: **Crazy Medical Stories**

This is a work of fiction. Unless otherwise stated – all names, characters, businesses, places, events, locales, and incidents in this book are the product of either the author's imagination or are used in a fictitious manner. Any resemblance to actual persons, living or dead, or actual events is purely coincidental.

ISBN: 978-1-7361598-4-2 (Paperback)

ISBN: 978-1-7361598-5-9 (EBook)

Second Edition 2021.

Credits:

Book Cover and Formatting by: farhanshahid101

Obsidian Wolf Publishing

PO Box 1086 Salem, UT 84653

Contents

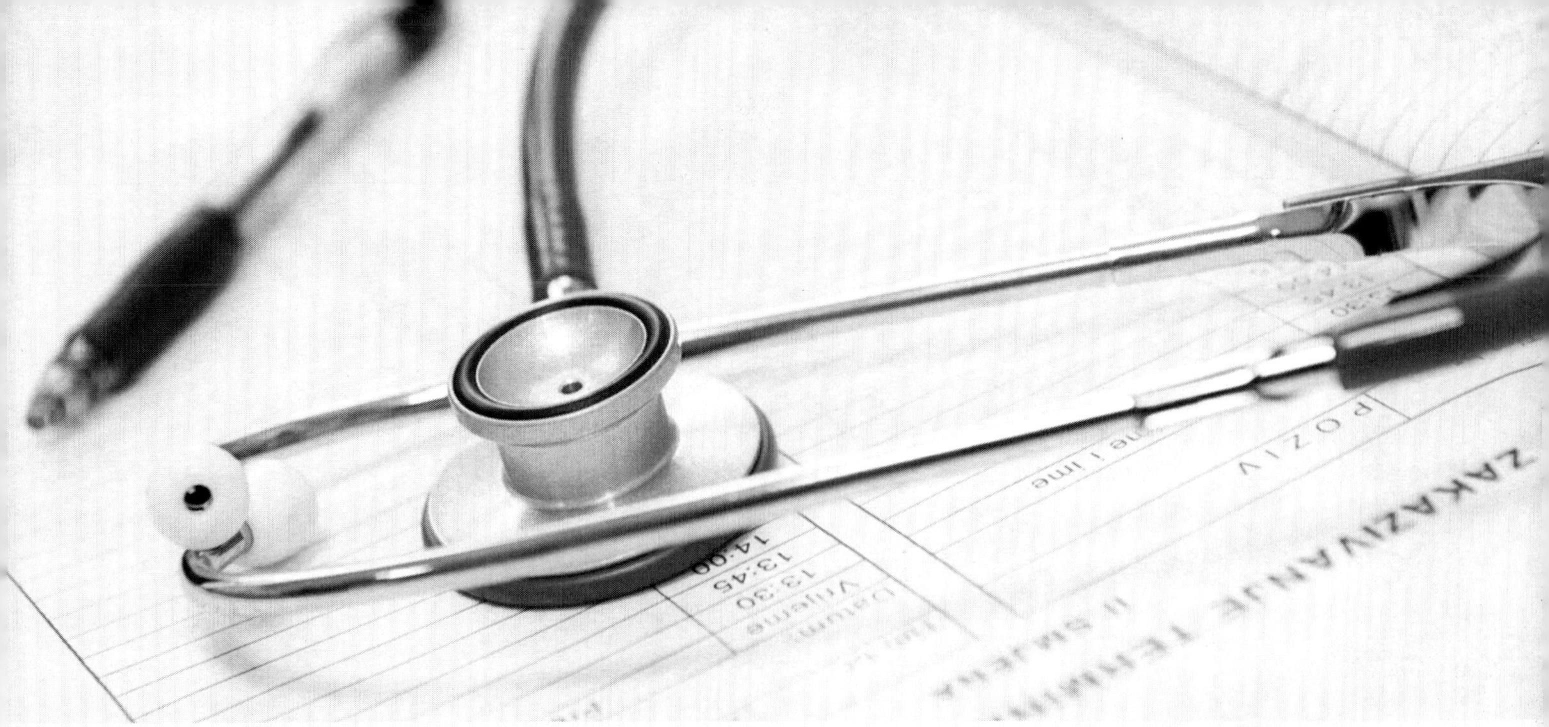

Introduction

Crazy Medical Stories: Tales of the Exam Room – *Volume 1* is designed first and foremost to make you laugh, cry, or even attempt to shock you. Every medical person in the world will have plenty of incredible stories to tell you - if you are willing to listen. This book is very much the same.

Our stories come from a variety of different medical professionals and many different areas of medicine. Each story has a different level of truth, and some stories have been combined. Much of the nature and the specifics of each medical story have been changed or altered. This is not intended to deceive but to protect the individual or individuals involved. This could include location, injury, storyline, and much more.

Again, this is a fictional piece and is largely for instruction and entertainment. Our goal is to allow you to see into the world of medicine and some of the bizarre encounters that have happened. We are not trying to poke fun at anyone. If your story happens to line up exactly with ours, trust me – we are not that good, and it's probably more of a coincidence. There are some medical truths and teachings that have been added for the readers' benefit.

Feel free to Join us for additional medical stories at: examroomtales.com

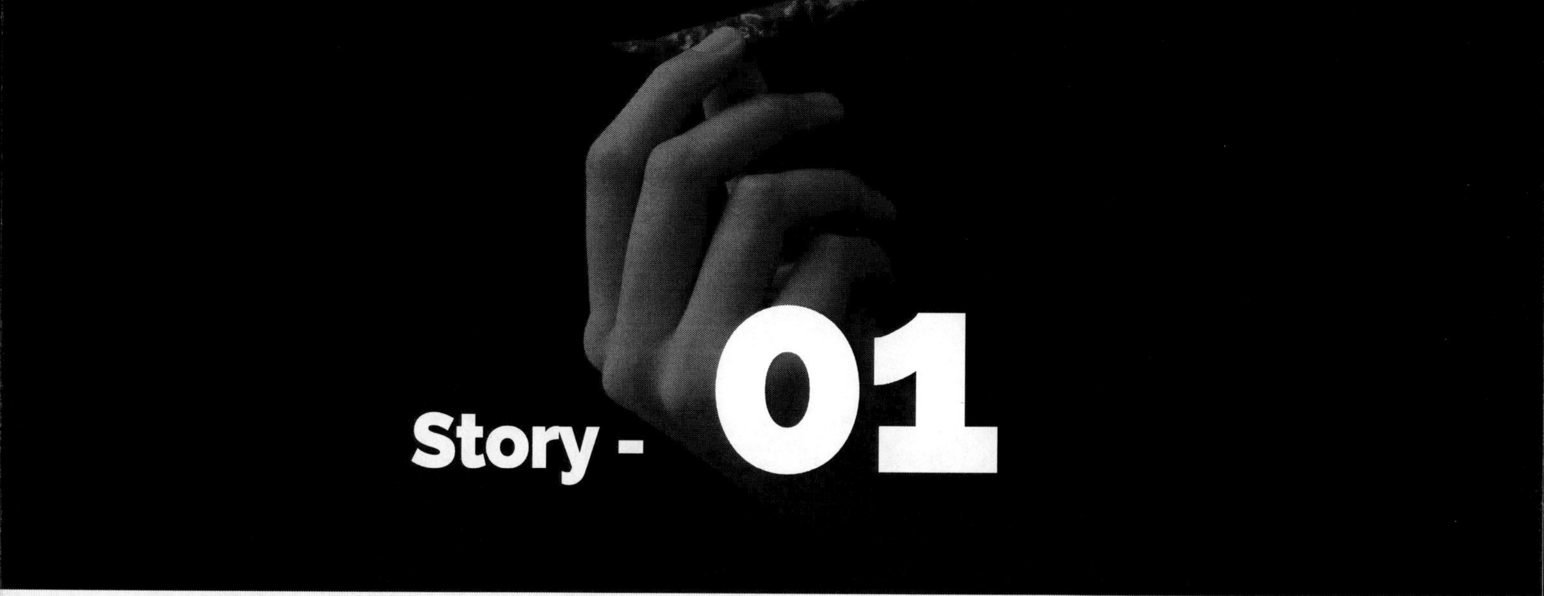

Tearing of the Esophagus from a Pepper

Imagine eating the hottest thing you've ever had in your life? What would that be? Salsa, Jerk Chicken, Kimchi jjigae, red chilis, or something else.

Research shows that each of us processes spicy foods differently, and that is why there is such a vastly different reaction to foods. And even the same person has some days where they can eat a vast amount of spicy foods, yet, another day, their response is far different.

This medical story comes to us from eating one of the hottest peppers in the world. Ghost Peppers have a "measured" heat of more than 1 million Scoville heat units. A jalapeno is measured around 5,000. It has been shown that a single seed can cause severe burning in the mouth for over thirty minutes.

In 2016, a 47-year-old man from California had an experience far different than he wanted or could have ever imagined. At a local restaurant, he was given a puree of Ghost peppers placed on top of a hamburger as part of an eating contest.

He began eating without a single concern except for his time on how fast he would finish the burger. He reportedly ate the entire thing, not a small feat. Quickly, because of the heat, he began guzzling water. In all, he drank six full glasses. Suddenly, after drinking the water, he began to vomit and retch violently. This continued, and soon, he was unable to stop vomiting. An ambulance was called, and he was rushed to the emergency room in San Francisco because he couldn't stop vomiting.

He was admitted to the hospital and sent for further evaluation. He underwent a CT scan of the chest. This specialized evaluation process showed that his esophagus was torn, and his left lung had collapsed. These were serious concerns, and the man was rushed in for surgery.

This story was reported by the Journal of Emergency Medicine, where it indicated that the man had a 1-inch tear in the esophagus. This allowed for food, onions, puree, bile, and water to settle around the lung, causing it to collapse. The surgery repaired the esophagus and helped treat the lung collapse. As a result of the injury and surgery, he was placed on a feeding tube for several weeks.

The patient suffered from a "Spontaneous Esophageal Rupture" or Boerhaave Syndrome. This is a very rare condition and is caused by violent vomiting and retching. It can be fatal in anywhere from 20-40 percent of the cases though it is not seen that often.

In this man's case, he was required to spend more than three weeks in the hospital before he was released. He kept a feeding tube in place until the lung and esophagus healed. It was expected that he would make a full recovery. I am pretty sure he will think twice before eating a ghost pepper again.

Without treatment, the condition would have proven to be fatal.

SOURCE

The Journal of Emergency Medicine:

Esophageal Rupture After Ghost Pepper Ingestion

https://www.jem-journal.com/article/S0736-4679(16)30256-6/pdf

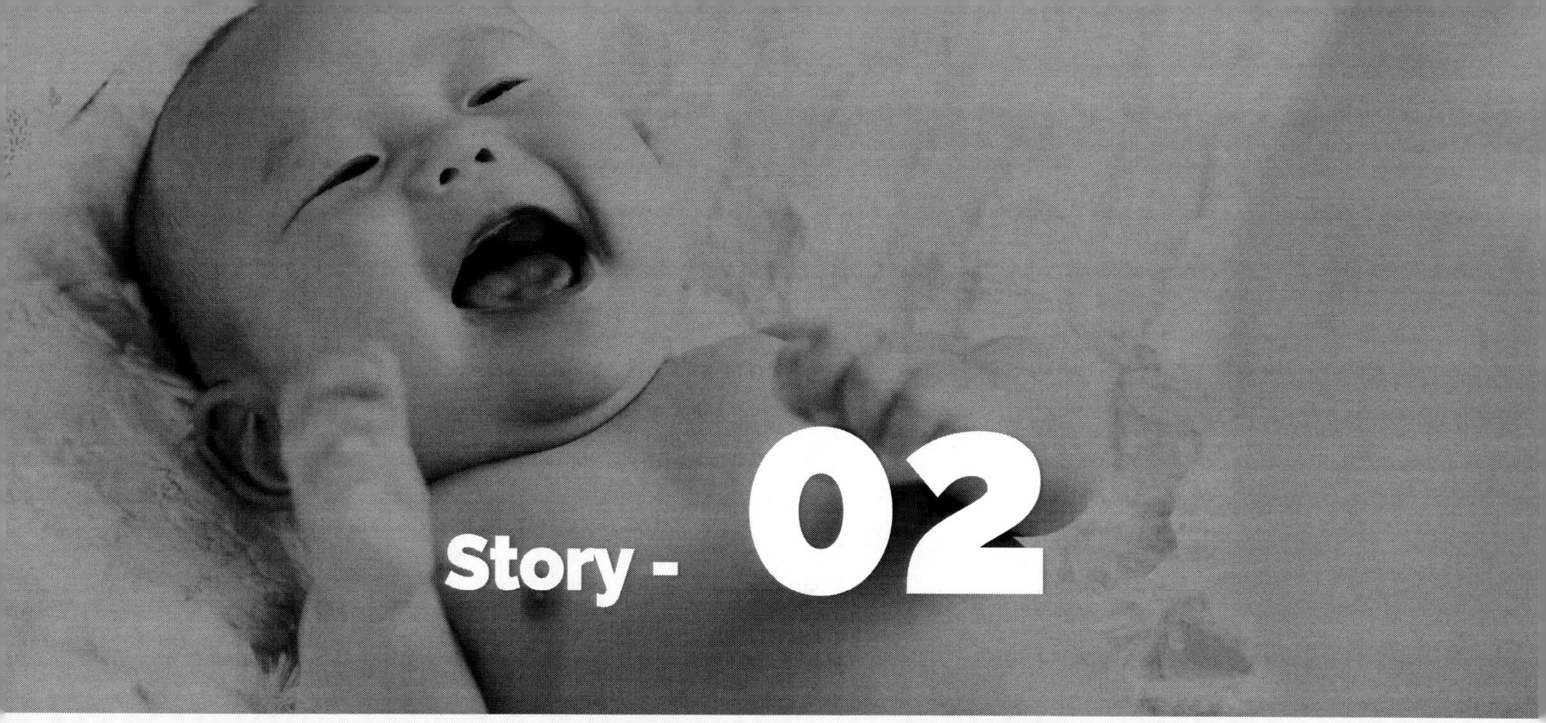

What Are You Feeding Your 6-Month Old?

A 22-year-old woman who was a first-time mom came into the clinic for a six-month check-up for her baby girl. We started with the general questions that are asked and answered. This process is to see if there have been any problems, changes, or general concerns from the family. It also gives the medical staff a good insight into how the mother or father is doing.

I had seen Mrs. Franklin a few times before. Those visits were often quick, with very few questions asked. Over the past few months, I was mildly surprised by this as often for first-time moms, and I get a hundred questions about anything you can imagine. I guessed that she had older siblings or friends that had children.

During this visit, Mrs. Franklin started by saying that the baby was doing pretty well. She assured me that the baby - Julia - was sleeping through the night. She would wake a few times during the night for feeding. Bottle-feeding and breastfeeding were taking place regularly. She indicated that she and her husband change diapers several times throughout the day. Overall, they had seen more movement, smiles, and the beginnings of a personality. They indicated they were delighted.

There did not seem to be any problems with nutrition, growth, breastfeeding, changing the diaper, or anything else. Overall, the mom had only a few generic questions about health and some of the 6-month milestones.

I learned that Julia was able to roll over without any problems. She could stand without support against the couch or similar. She was an active child who loved to play with toys and often placed objects in her mouth. She was able to babble with some unrecognizable words. She hadn't started crawling yet, but Mrs. Franklin thought this would be happening soon.

The physical exam of the child was normal. No concerning weight loss and normal head size and length were noted. I saw no obvious problems, pains, or other issues during the exam. Julia was attentive, curious, with bright blue eyes and brown hair.

We moved into the food portion of the discussion. Julia had a real interest in food. She would open her mouth when food approached her mouth. She tolerated puree foods but really loved her bottle. Her mother had tried some pureed food with only a single ingredient, such as carrots, apples, and pears.

This was when I asked to see Julia's bottle. Mrs. Franklin pulled out the bottle, and I was shocked to see that it was half-filled with chocolate milk.

I exclaimed, "Mrs. Franklin. Remember us talking a few months ago that we can't give Julia cow's milk until after the age of one. This includes chocolate milk."

"I completely remember."

"So, why are you giving her chocolate milk?"

"I've never given Julia chocolate milk or any cow's milk for that matter. I'm a staunch believer in avoiding milk and other dairy products. I've read up on the problems of giving milk. I want Julia to be the healthiest possible."

I lifted up the baby bottle, showing her, and said, "This looks an awful lot like chocolate milk."

She smiled kindly at me and replied, "Don't worry, Doctor, that's not chocolate milk. That is an iced coffee. Julia totally loves them."

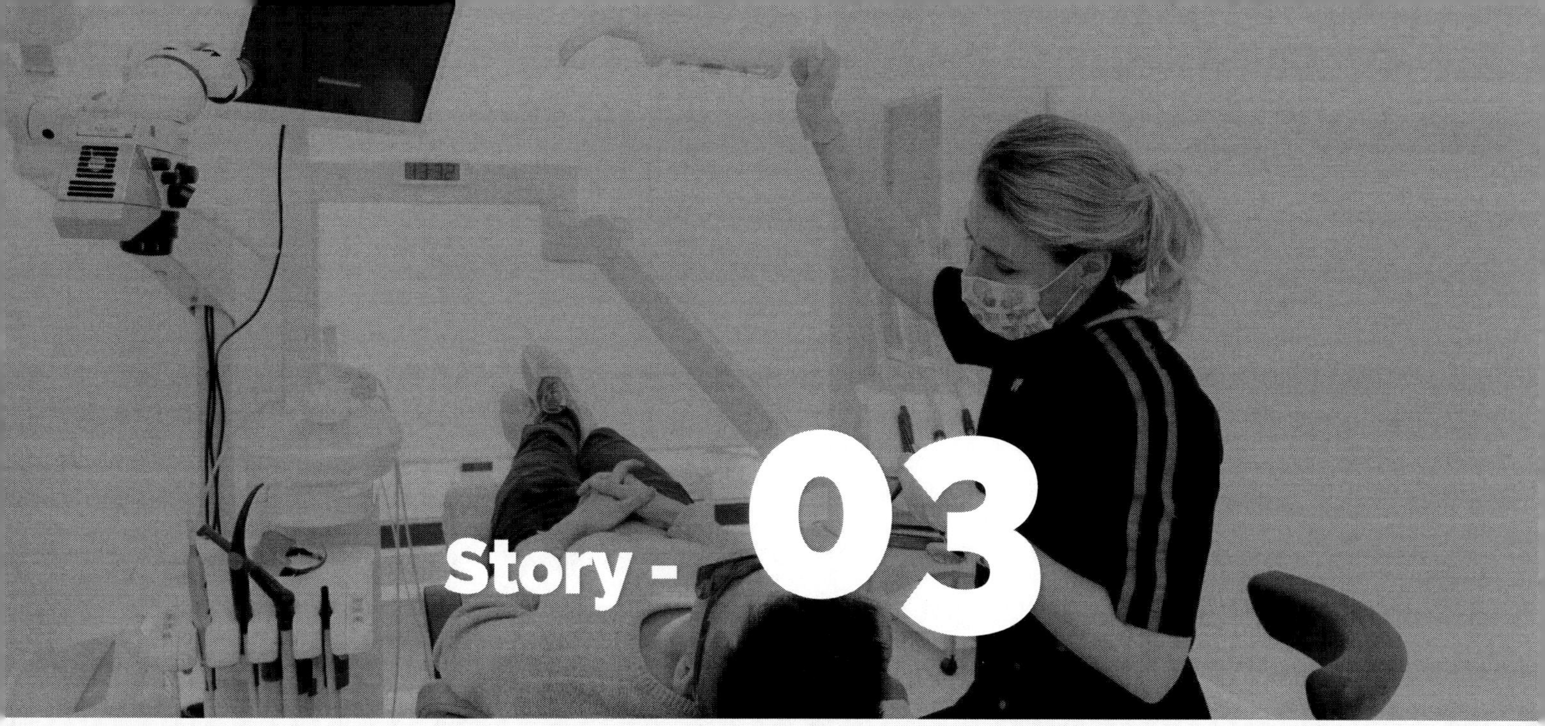

An Agitated Patient Demanding Medications

My medical assistant added a patient to my schedule after berating my office staff for over an hour, despite not having an appointment for the day. Our clinic keeps a few open appointments just in case this happens. Even after my MAs brought her to her room, she continued to complain and went as far as to threaten some of my staff. She refused to give the nurse, or anyone else, more information about what was going on or why she needed to be seen. In fact, she had never been seen in my office before. The only thing that was written on the chart was: Patient wants a refill of her medications.

Entering the exam room, I was halfway through my schedule for the day. The patient was seated and staring at her phone. She appeared to be a mess. She was anxious, pale, and shaking. Tears were running down her face. I immediately felt compassion for her. It is my experience that patients often go through challenging things. By the time I see them, they've struggled or suffered for days, weeks, and even longer.

I tried to set aside my initial feelings of defending my staff and tried to picture what this lady must be going through. She was seeing a medical provider for the first time. We were practically strangers to her, asking her to tell us difficult information. It can't be easy. Some of the questions that are asked might be embarrassing. That's the point, though. You're telling a relative stranger your problems and hoping they can fix them.

The first few questions I asked were pretty basic with background, medications, and surgical histories. This lady was pleasant, and she answered each of them fully, with plenty of information and without reservation. Despite her answers, she was still in quite a bit of distress.

After finishing the initial questions, I asked, "So, what brings you into the office today?"

"I've gotten myself into quite a mess. I've done things with people that I'm not proud of. Sometimes, you have to do what you have to do. But I heard that you could help me."

"This is the right place. We can fix most messes, and you can even come out better on the opposite side."

The lady smiled for the first time. "That sounds good. Thank you for understanding."

She stood and walked towards the door. "So, you'll call in the prescription that I need."

"Wait," I said quickly. "I need a little more information than that. And we might have to do some testing, just to make sure." I have to admit that at this point, I thought I had narrowed down why she was here to a few possible choices.

"What kind of testing?"

"A urine sample, pregnancy test, and some blood work. We have a lab here that can facilitate all of this."

"Great," she said. "No one's ever done that before."

"You've had similar problems before?"

"A few times. Never this bad, though."

"Who treated you before?"

"I can't remember. Usually, my friends."

This answer was a little confusing, but I pushed on. "How many times?"

"No more than three or four times."

"This is what we call risky behavior."

"I guess I can see that."

I continued, "There are significant risks associated that can led to more serious medical problems."

"I totally agree. Why do you think that I came in when I did? I felt that it had become an emergency. Do you think you can put refills on the prescription? I won't abuse it myself. I'm not into that."

At this comment, a second red flag emerged in my mind. Sitting down, I said, "What prescription would you like me to write?"

"Hydrocodone with Tylenol. I don't think I need more than sixty."

"You want me to prescribe you, Lortab?"

"That's what I need. I knew that you were the only one who would understand."

"Why exactly do you need it? Did you have a recent injury or a chronic issue?" I began searching her chart. She hadn't mentioned anything similar in the first set of questions. I asked, "Have you been prescribed this before?"

"As I said, I usually get this from a friend, but he won't answer my calls. But don't worry, I really don't use them myself."

"Why exactly do you need them?"

"It's complicated."

I stared at her in disbelief. I said, "Prescribing a narcotic is a serious thing. I can't just order them based on this little information. I need to know what's going on."

She licked her lips and said, "Look. I've been selling Lortab to some of my friends and neighbors for the last several months. I sort of ran out of them a few weeks ago, and I didn't have a ton of them left. Half the neighborhood was asking for them. So, I began giving out Tylenol instead. Both pills are white and similar. But I think a few of my neighbors caught on. They're stopping by my house later tonight, and I need to have the real stuff. They are threatening me. Maybe you should make it ninety. That should get me through the next few days."

"Are you crazy? You can't come into a doctor's office and ask for Lortab to sell. That's illegal. I should call the police."

"No, it's not. It's no illegal to sell medication. That's what the pharmacies do all the time. I've heard you can get them online or from Canada or Mexico. It's only illegal to sell Heroin, Meth, or Cocaine. I know my rights."

Standing, I said, "No. You're mistaken. Are you trying to joke with me? This can't be serious."

Defensively she responded, "I'm not doing anything wrong, and I'm helping my family."

"You need to leave right now, or I am going to call the police. This is your last warning."

"Chill out. I'm leaving." She walked to the door, stopped, and turned around. She said, "You're so confusing. Before, you were willing to help me. You told me about labs and medications. What changed?"

"That was when I thought you had an STD."

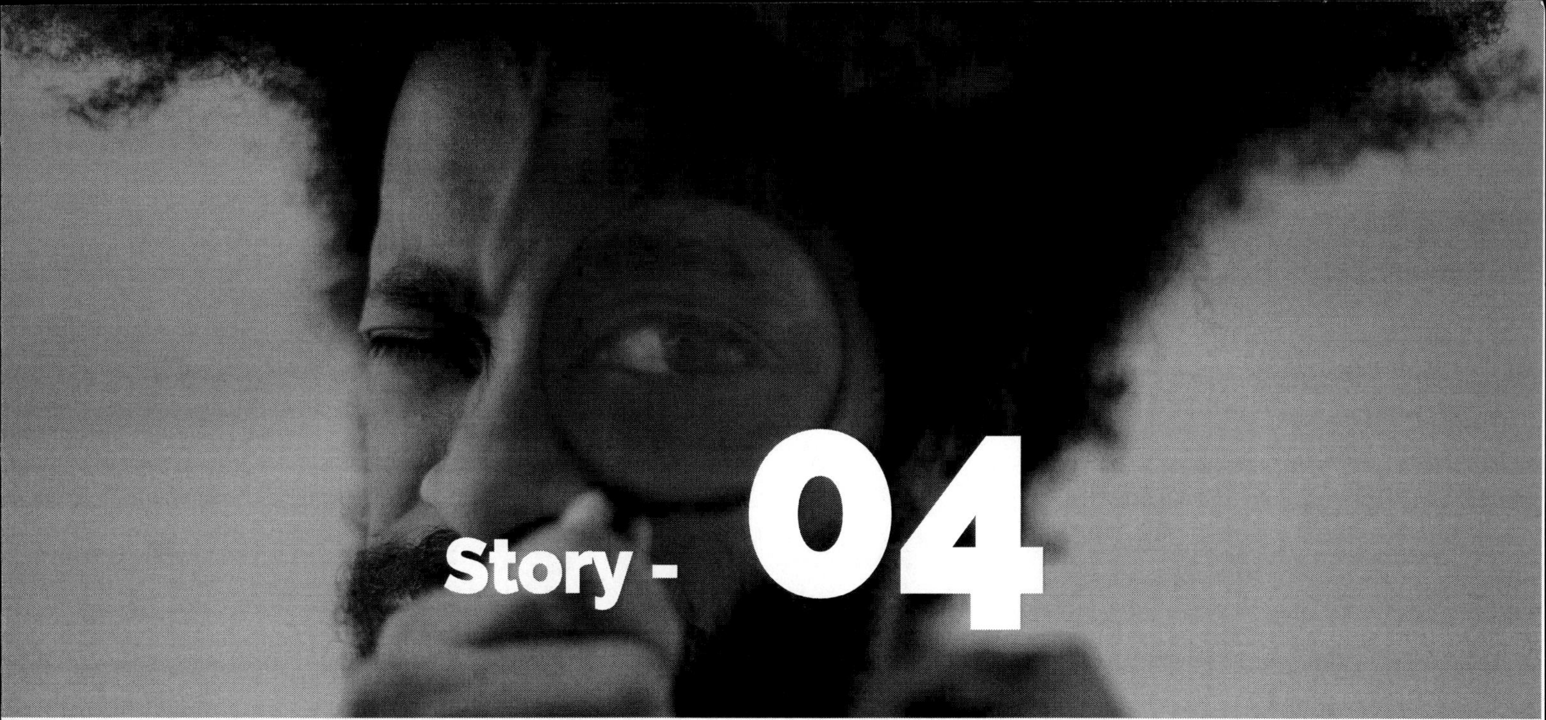

Story - 04

A Self Injury to The Eye

On our medical unit, it seems that when you're called to the same patient's room two or three times in a short amount of time unexpectedly, then one of three things is likely occurring. 1.) The patient is really in need of something. 2.) The patient might be overstating their needs. 3.) The patient intends to or about to do something crazy - so be prepared.

One night, last year, around three in the morning, this type of experience is precisely what I found myself involved in. I was on the unit for a graveyard shift, and it was just a few minutes past midnight. It was my third of five shifts in a row, and I was called to the room of a female patient that was on medical observation. She'd been on the unit for about five days. She had been recently started on some new medications, and the staff was seeing some improvement in her behavior.

The first call was for a very typical complaint. She indicated that she was having a hard time going to the bathroom. This can happen with some mental health medications. I gave her some Milk of Magnesia, intended to help clean out the bowels.

This was my first interaction with this patient for the night. I found her pleasant but slightly odd. In where I work, this is not unusual. We have a lot of challenging patients.

The second time I was called to her room, not fifteen minutes later, turned out to be far more suspicious and concerning. The patient was now suddenly paranoid. She was out of her bed, looking around, completely frazzled. She was convinced that someone had opened her door, peeked in, and was staring at her while she slept. I reminded her that I had just visited her, gave her some medications, not fifteen minutes previously.

Apparently, she'd completely forgotten about our initial encounter. She was convinced that she'd never received any medications and that someone was stalking her. I tried to reassure her, but she was anything but satisfied. I searched her closet, her bathroom, and even under her bed, trying to soothe her.

"Nope," I told her. "There's no one here."

"He was staring at me. I think I saw a knife in his hand."

I wasn't sure what to say next. After a moment, I added, "Well, he's gone. I'll have security posted outside your room to make sure no one comes back."

"Oh, fantastic."

She stared at me with absolute relief stretched across her face. She added, "Thank you so much. You saved my life. I'll be better now."

"My pleasure. I'll come back and check on you in the next hour or so."

"Thank you! Thank you! Thank you!"

Pulling up her covers, she smiled and closed her eyes. I quickly left her room. I hadn't taken more than twenty steps towards my desk when an ear-piercing scream erupted from her room. I sprinted back, and when I opened the door, I witnessed something I'd never seen before. My patient was hitting herself in the stomach–one punch, then two, then three.

I sprinted in screaming, "Stop. What's wrong?"

She immediately stopped punching her stomach. But as she looked up at me, I could tell that something was seriously wrong. Her hand groped at her own face, and she began scratching vigorously. She was mumbling, "Try to see me the F*#$ now." She started laughing hysterically.

I yelled into my radio, "Crisis team to room 212".

I wasn't sure if I should try to restrain her from hurting herself. That was when I noticed that she was trying to scratch out her own eye. I watched in horror as one finger sunk into the flesh just above her right eye. In terror and in slow motion, I watched as she began pulling at her eye. I screamed, "Stop," and ran forward.

As I reached her bed, the sound I heard will be something that I'll never forget. I grabbed both of her hands and pulled them away. But it was too late.

Additional staff arrived a moment later, and it didn't take long for her to be restrained and sedated. She'd severely scratched her face, and there was a fair amount of blood. Her eye was still attached, but it was just out of her socket - still connected by the nerve - the optic nerve.

I'll never forget the disturbing image of her eye just dangling there. She was immediately transferred to the local hospital, where she was able to see a specialist. They were able to place the eye back in the socket with only minimal long-term damage. She has some vision loss and blurriness, but it was far better than what it could've been.

That night, for whatever reason, my patient was in an awful place, and she made matters worse. She was started on heavier medications and therapy, and over time she improved dramatically. Sometimes mental health can create a situation that we don't always understand what someone else is thinking. It was undoubtedly a learning moment for me.

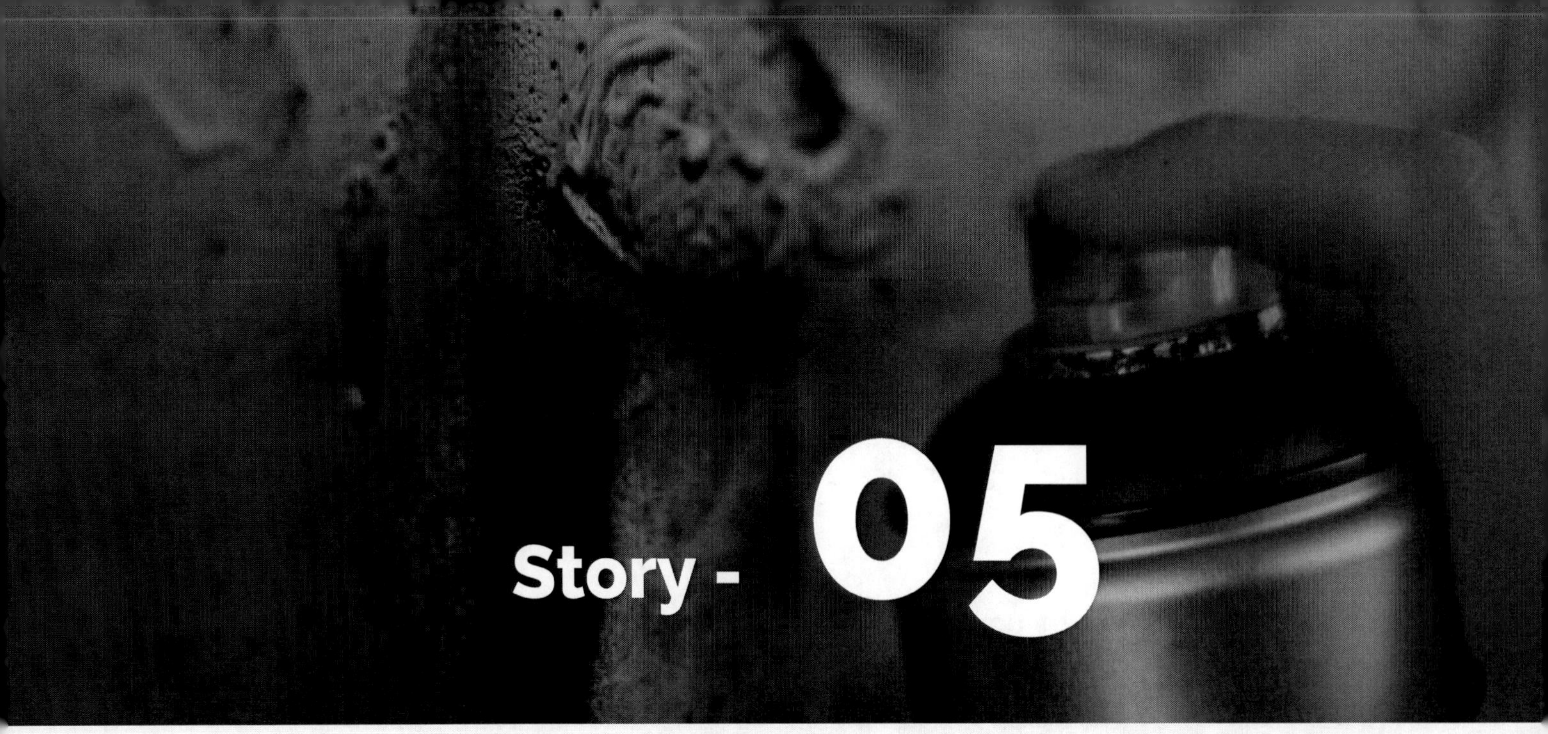

Story - 05

Seizure Caused by Huffing Paint

An ambulance pulled up to the entrance of an emergency room with its lights flashing. The back door opened, and two EMTs jumped out the back. They begin unloading their patient, who was strapped to the backboard. The patient started screaming, and the sounds echoed around the corridor. Soon several medical staff was running in their direction. It took more than one individual to tighten him to the stretcher, protecting himself.

The man screamed, "Help me. I'm going to have another seizure and die! Someone help me."

It didn't take long for Nurse Vicky, the charge nurse, to take control of the situation. She was able to get the patient to stop screaming and to focus. She asked, "What's your name?"

"David Sanders. Please don't let me have another seizure. It's the worst pain I've ever experienced."

"We're going to do the best we can," Nurse Vicky assured him. "You're safe now."

In a pleading voice, David added, "Please help me."

"Can you tell me what happened?"

"I had a terrible seizure at work. I was working on the oil rig and went to get some equipment. When I went inside a shed, something happened, but I can't remember. My coworker splashed some water on my face, and I woke up. He told me an ambulance was on the way."

"Have you ever had a seizure before?"

"I don't think so."

"When did this happen?"

"About thirty minutes ago, but I am not really sure."

By this time, the medical staff had wheeled David into the hospital and into an exam room. Nurse Vicky asked, "What kind of seizure did you have? Why did it happen?"

"I've no idea. That's why I'm here. I feel another one coming on. This one is going to be so bad that I could die."

Doctor Stevens stepped into the room. He was quickly updated on the patient's complaints and condition.

After the introductions, Doctor Stevens asked, "Have you ever hit your head or had a high fever that led to a seizure?"

"I don't know, man. Not that I can remember."

David Sanders' body suddenly became rigid, and he started shaking. He was flopping everywhere, his arms hitting his chest repeatedly. All-the-while he was yelling, "Don't leave me. This is bad! Please give me something to make it stop."

Doctor Steven's shouted, "Start an IV and let's get some lab work. Prepare for a brain MRI."

"Thank you, Doctor," Mr. Sanders mouthed as Doctor Stevens and Nurse Vicky exited the room.

Out in the waiting area, Doctor Stevens and Nurse Vicky searched for Jared Finter, the coworker that had found him, and had accompanied him to the hospital. He was getting a cup of coffee in the small cafeteria.

They began asking questions, trying to better identify the cause.

After answering a few questions, Jared Finter asked, "Is David going to be alright?"

"I'm sure he will. But we'll watch him for a few hours and make sure all his blood work comes back normal. We will scan his brain; it's called an MRI machine. It will help us detect if anything seriously wrong is happening."

After a moment, Doctor Stevens nodded, and Nurse Vicky asked, "Did you find him, with that ring of paint around his nose and mouth?"

"Um…" Jared appeared slightly uncomfortable, glancing away.

"Yes. He's often huffing paint, in fact, a few times a week, but this time, he was in there for much longer than usual."

"How did he look when you found him?" asked Doctor Stevens.

"Foaming around his mouth, and he was shaking something fierce."

"How long did it last?"

"Maybe thirty seconds."

"Thank you," Doctor Stevens said. "We are going to find a way to help your friend."

After getting the blood work results and the MRI, Doctor Stevens returned to David's room. He was resting comfortably, his eyes closed. "David. You have a problem."

"Am I going to die?"

"Well. That depends on you."

"What do you mean?"

"Your blood work and your brain MRI came back normal. But I think you know exactly why this happened."

"I had a seizure."

"Most likely. But the essential point to discuss, is what was the cause of your seizure?"

"That's what I need to know."

Doctor Stevens continued, "You're at a larger risk of brain damage and seizures when you're huffing paint. Your coworkers are aware of your addiction, and this time, it resulted in a simple seizure. This is a very serious problem. Huffing paint is dangerous."

"I don't think that's my problem. I'm here to see you because I had a seizure. I don't huff."

Lifting a mirror, Doctor Stevens pointed to the dried paint ring around his nose and mouth. He added, "The evidence says otherwise. You have a huffing problem. Huffing can cause seizures, and one day, it may kill you."

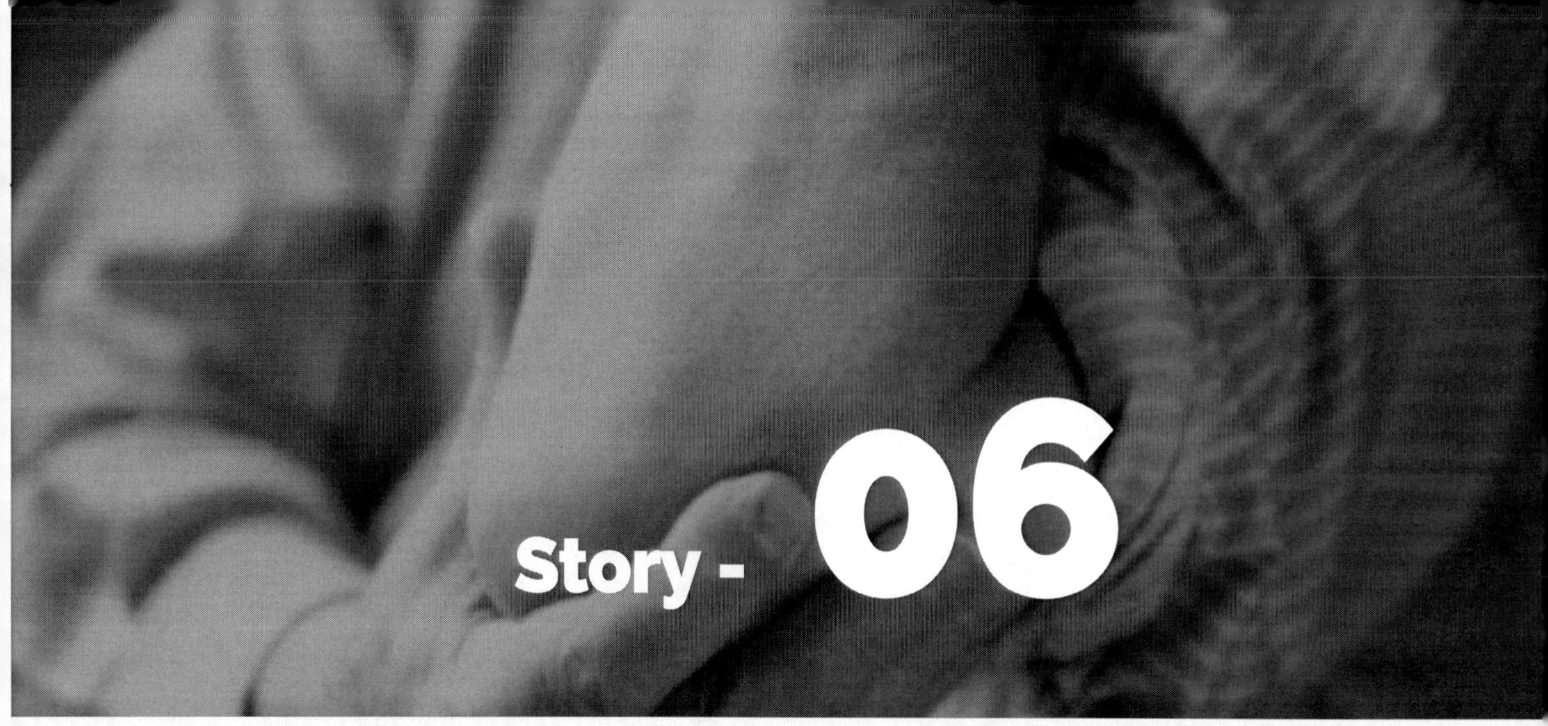

I Can See Bone and Metal Sticking out of your Elbow

Anytime you have an open wound, you are at risk of getting an infection. This could be from a bite, a cut in the skin, a car accident, significant trauma, or anything else. When that open wound doesn't heal the way that it should and it remains open, there is an increased risk of infection and potentially sustaining life-altering problems in the future.

This story starts when the patient, Mike Rigby, was skateboarding, and he fell and injured his elbow. He knew it was injured, but he hoped it wasn't anything serious. He had an abrasion but couldn't get a real good look at it. Mike decided to clean it out the best he could and wrapped a large ACE wrap with gauze and hope for the best.

At first, because of the pain, he was reluctant to move his arm. The pain was definitely worse at night when he slept on his arm. Over the next few days, the pain continued getting worse and worse. Around day five, he tried to straighten his arm but couldn't. By this time, he was starting to have some fever and chills and felt nauseous. He became concerned that this was more than just a scrape of the skin.

Two days later, he finally decided to go to the emergency room, where they did an X-ray, and it was determined that the severity of the injury would require surgery. In fact, he had a broken elbow and an infection. The surgeon placed a metal plate and some screws into the bones of the elbow. He was placed in a soft cast and given some antibiotics.

Once home, he was limited on how much he could lift and move. The first few weeks, Mike felt horrible. It took several more weeks for the healing process to be completed. Afterward, physical therapy was required, and it seemed that he was healing well.

Several weeks later, Mike was out partying and having a good time. As the story goes, he was drinking quite a bit. He was dancing and acting crazy. At one point, he slipped and fell onto the ground. It didn't hurt, really, but his elbow started to bleed.

Some of his friends noticed the bleeding first, and they put a bandage on his arm. It took a few gauze wraps for the bleeding to stop. He crashed at the house, and the next morning he headed home, almost oblivious to the elbow injury. The next day was the first day that he removed the initial dressing. It was still slightly bleeding. He showered and placed another gauze bandage on the arm.

Mike thought it took about a week for a scab to form on the elbow. By this time, he was feeling much better. The pain had resolved, and he could bend his arm without any limitations.

About 2-3 weeks later, he was required to get a physical exam for a new job. He denied any medical issues or complaints. During the physical exam, the medical provider quickly noticed several problems with the elbow. Mike had an open wound the size of a quarter. The skin was pulled back, and the metal plate and two screws were clearly visible. Even a portion of the bone was sticking out.

When asked, Mike recounted the story of falling, but he reluctantly admitted that he never took the time to examine the elbow. He'd been confident that it would heal on its own and really didn't think much more about it.

The doctor said, "We need to be worried about an infection. We should probably get some blood work."

"I've already done that before," Mike insisted. "Can't we just wrap it?"

"This type of infection would be much more serious than the one you had before."

"Can't I just soak it in hydrogen peroxide and keep it bandaged?"

"Not this time."

Mike was admitted to the hospital again, and additional tests were ordered. He hated the fact that he needed more blood work, X-rays, and a CT. When the doctor overseeing him came back with the news that he needed another surgery, Mike was pissed.

At first, he refused the surgery.

Doctor Phan explained, "The bone around the metal is now infected. If we close the skin or it heals, the infection won't be going away. We need to cut out some of the bone."

"Are you serious?" Mike asked.

"Completely," Dr. Phan replied.

This time, they had to remove all the metal, screws, and some of the bone. The surgeon had to scrape the bone to get rid of the infection. A second, larger metal plate was inserted. It took weeks and weeks for the bone and skin to heal.

A year later, Mike has some range of motion loss and some nerve damage because of the infection and the second surgery. Even with those problems, it could've been much worse.

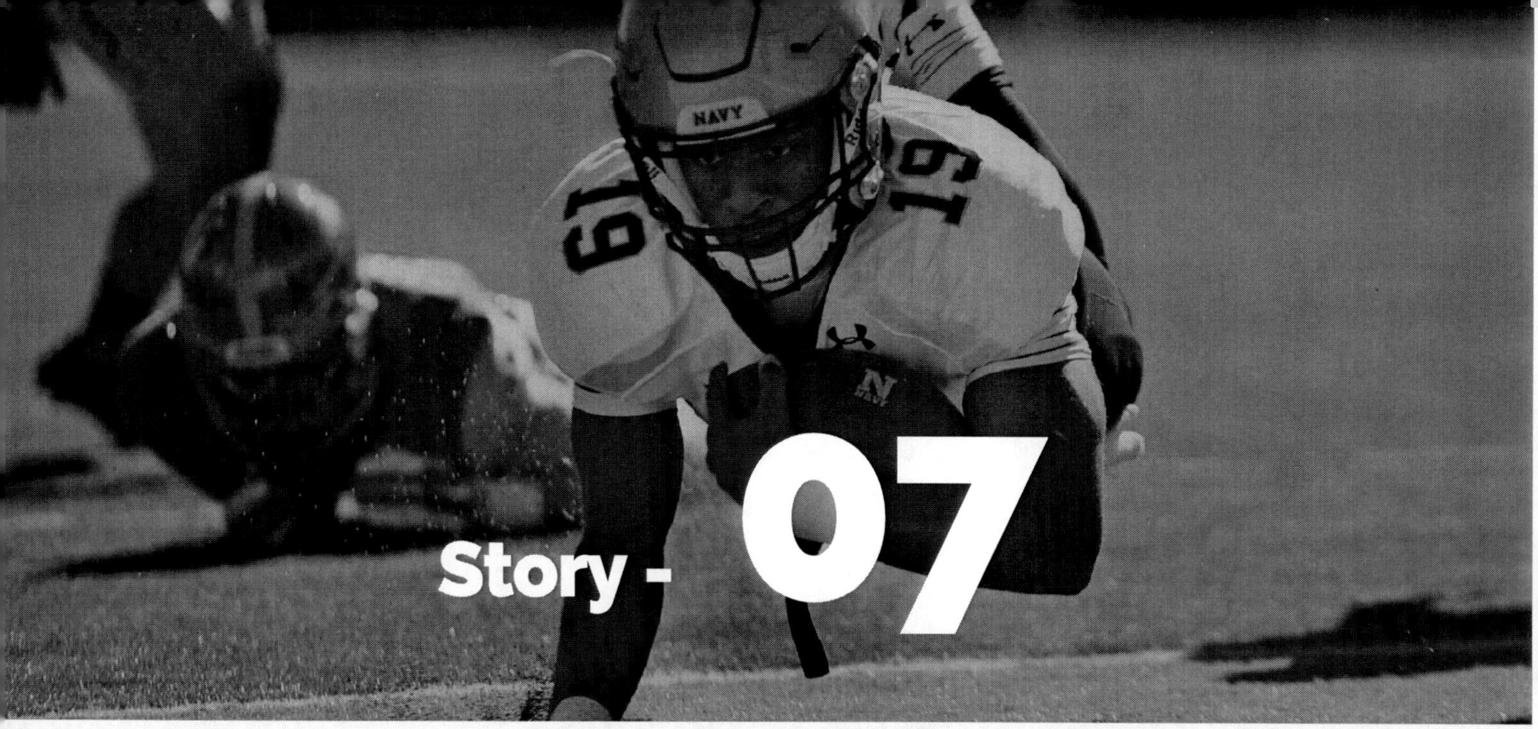

The Superbowl Makes Some Men Stupid

Recently I was working on the day of the Superbowl. I am not a big football fan, and this year, I didn't even know who was playing. My shift was going great; I mean, for a Sunday, it was quiet and calm. I was able to work on getting caught up with my paperwork and even found time to review some of my continuing education credits.

I voiced my happiness to some of the other staff, and the attending doctor warned me to be ready. He said, "Once the game is over, everything will change."

He was not lying.

Fifteen minutes before the game ended, the waiting line for the emergency room tripled. People started pouring in, and we were slammed for a few hours. Most of the cases were simple enough – chest pain from eating spicy food and anxiety from their team not winning. Most of the injures and medical problems could be loosely tied to the game or worse for waiting to come to the hospital until the game was over.

Two patients, arriving five minutes apart, seemed to know each other extremely well. When the first ambulance arrived, the male patient was in a tremendous amount of pain. He had a lower leg injury consistent with a fall. He was screaming, and they were having a difficult time controlling his pain. That gentleman wasn't my patient. The second one, who arrived five minutes later, was my patient.

To my knowledge, the two men weren't related, but they kept screaming and yelling at each other from one exam room to another. They were hostile and demeaning, and it was hard to get anything done.

When I stepped into my patient's room, he was finishing a string of profanities that made me blush. It turned out that he also had a lower extremity injury. After the X-rays were done, it appeared that he almost had the same exact injury as his friend.

I took the second X-ray and compared it to the first just to make sure there wasn't a mix-up. I peeked in on the first patient and found him to be riling in pain with the same leg injury. It was unsettling.

Returning to my patient, we set off to control his pain and help him feel comfortable. He had a significant leg fracture on his left leg that would require surgery. He was second in line for surgery, and he would have an hour before they would take him upstairs.

Once he was comfortable, I began talking with him. My patient was Derrick.

I asked, "It's remarkable to see the same injury in two different patients. I can't tell you anything specific about the other patient. Will you explain what is happening?"

He said, "Oh, you must be talking about that a**hole, Greg."

"I really can't confirm a name or share someone else's medical information."

"No worries," he said. "I know that you are talking about Greg."

"What happened?" I asked.

"Football and money."

"Are you telling me that this is about the Superbowl?"

Derrick said, "Exactly. My team won, and I'm so beyond excited that it happened. It's been twenty years since they won. I didn't think it would ever happen."

I replied, "Um...?"

Derrick continued, "You see, Greg over there, bet on the other team. He put down quite a bit of money. He placed the bet when his team was ahead by a few touchdowns."

"I guess Greg's team started not doing so well."

Chuckling, he added, "Horrible, in fact. My team ended up winning. Greg owes me a lot of money."

"That still doesn't explain your injuries."

"We got into this fight. I was pushing him around a little bit. He knows that if he places a bet, he needs to pay."

I asked, "Did you hurt him?"

He said, "Of course not. Instead of paying me, that idiot tried to escape by jumping out my window, two stories above the ground."

My hand went to my mouth, shocked. I asked, "Then what happened to you?"

Shaking his head, he added, "I guess I'm even stupider. I wanted my money and followed him. I jumped out the same window to collect my money."

Both men went to surgery, requiring practically the same operation to fix their broken leg. They paid far more for their medical bills than any bet on a sports game. At least... I hope.

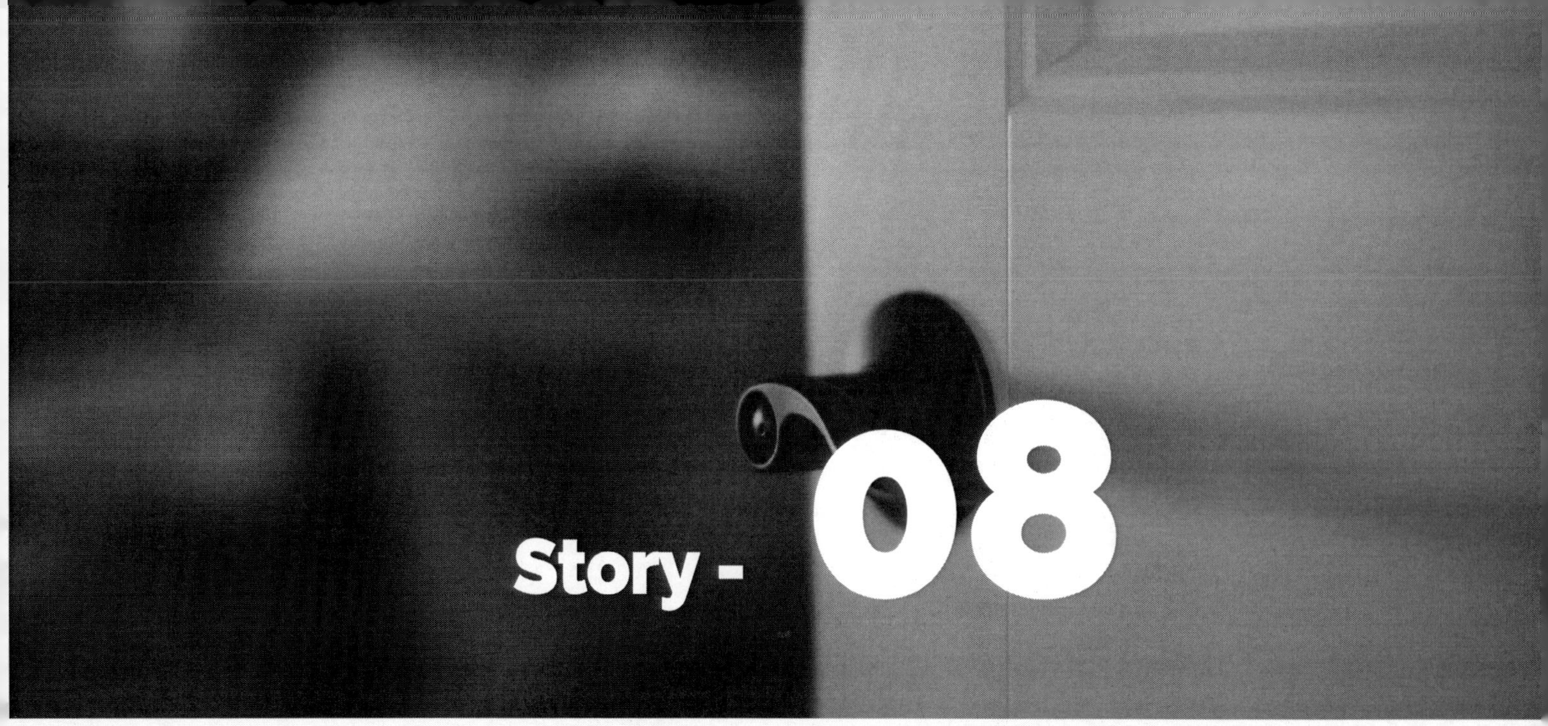

Home Health Disaster

I had been gone two weeks on vacation and returned to work at my home health job. My second patient of the day was one of my favorites. Jimmy Dallon was a 54-year-old male with Hypertension and Diabetes. This visit turned out to be one of the most bizarre of my career.

Although considered legally blind, Jimmy could still see the television and read a book using a giant magnifying glass. He was not allowed to drive. I had been working with him for two years. His wife had passed away five years previously, and he needed a nurse to come into his home twice a week to make sure that his oral medications were prepared and that he had the supplies needed for the week. Additionally, I helped around his apartment and checked him for any infections or other medical problems. I was more than happy to help in any way that I could.

When I arrived at Jimmy's apartment, I should've known something was wrong when he wasn't greeting me at the door or on the couch watching television. Two other newer nurses had filled in for me while I was gone. They didn't know Jimmy like I did and hadn't spent much time cleaning his apartment.

The apartment was a mess, and it smelled like a window hadn't been opened in two weeks. I quickly took a moment to check on Jimmy and found him sleeping in his bed. I then began cleaning the apartment, starting with the kitchen. There was a fair amount of spoiled food, and I cleaned out the fridge. Soon I was vacuuming and starting a load of laundry. It took an hour or a little longer, but soon things were looking better. I rarely did this much cleaning, but I felt bad for how bad Jimmy's apartment had become.

Jimmy lives in a downtown apartment in a larger city on the fifth floor. We have great public transportation like buses and such, but I need a car to get to my appointments quickly. After cleaning the kitchen, I returned to my car and grabbed some of the things I needed to get Jimmy ready for the week. I took out the trash with me as I was heading downstairs. When I came back upstairs, I grabbed his mail from the first floor. There was at least one week of mail inside his box. I started getting an uneasy feeling.

When I entered the apartment, the front room smelled so much better, but the same couldn't be said for Jimmy's room. His bathroom had gauze and other supplies, both used and new. His bathroom area had pills that were spilled on the floor. The area was a disaster area. This time, I didn't start cleaning and rushed to Jimmy's bedside to check on him.

Jimmy was sweating profusely, and his pulse was sky-high. I tried waking him, but he refused to open his eyes. I pulled back his covers and found that he had vomited and urinated all over his bed. It was not a pretty sight. Jimmy wore shorts and a t-shirt. The next thing I noticed was that his left foot was wrapped with an ace bandage. I can tell the difference between a nurse wrapping an area and when the patient or someone else does. This had not been done by a nurse.

I quickly placed a phone call to one of the nurses that had been here in the last few weeks. When she answered, she was unsurprised by the behavior of Mr. Dallon. She explained that he was pretty responsive initially, but then things got worse. She had been worried that his dementia was getting bad. He kept forgetting to put things away and what medications he was taking. I told her that Mr. Dallon didn't have significant dementia.

After I hung up the phone, I grabbed my glucometer from my bag and checked Jimmy's blood sugar. He was always well controlled on his two oral medications. I was shocked to see that his blood sugar reading read -Hi-.

Most of the time, you want a blood sugar below 100. In a Diabetic patient, you hope it's below 150 most of the time, especially if they are taking just oral medications. Mr. Dallon had never taken Insulin, but at this moment, that was exactly what he needed.

In the absence of an order for Insulin, Jimmy needed to go to the hospital, especially with his change in behavior. I began changing his shirt and shorts, and it took a while to change his clothes. The last thing I did was to start to remove the ACE bandage on his leg.

As I removed it, the smell in the room worsened significantly. There was some swelling of his leg, but the more concerning appearance was his foot. A large glob of toilet paper was stuck to his foot. I kept removing the tissues, and not long afterward, I realized that the tissue was continuing into a hole on the side of his foot. It turned out to be the worst thing I've ever seen.

If I could describe his foot, in hopes for you to understand, it was as if someone had taken a small ice cream scoop and scooped out the side of his foot. There was a three-inch hole in his foot. Mr. Dallon had been sticking toilet paper repeatedly into the hole. The smell of the dead tissue was sickening.

I immediately called an ambulance, and Mr. Dallon was transferred to the hospital. It turned out that he was in Diabetic Ketoacidosis or DKA, which is a serious risk for those with diabetes. This can be a life-threatening complication.

Additionally, he had an infection in his leg that had eventually gone to his bone. It took a few days to get his sugars under control and for him to start feeling better. However, a few days later, it was determined that he needed his leg amputated up to the knee. He stayed in the hospital for another few weeks to recover.

When he finally came home, I stopped by every day for two weeks. It took him a while to get used to the wheelchair and many other required changes. In speaking with him, he told me that he went into a fog for several days. He wasn't able to remember a lot of what happened.

He couldn't remember me coming into his room and changing him and calling an ambulance. He's back to normal now, as nice as ever. It was a terrifying incident.

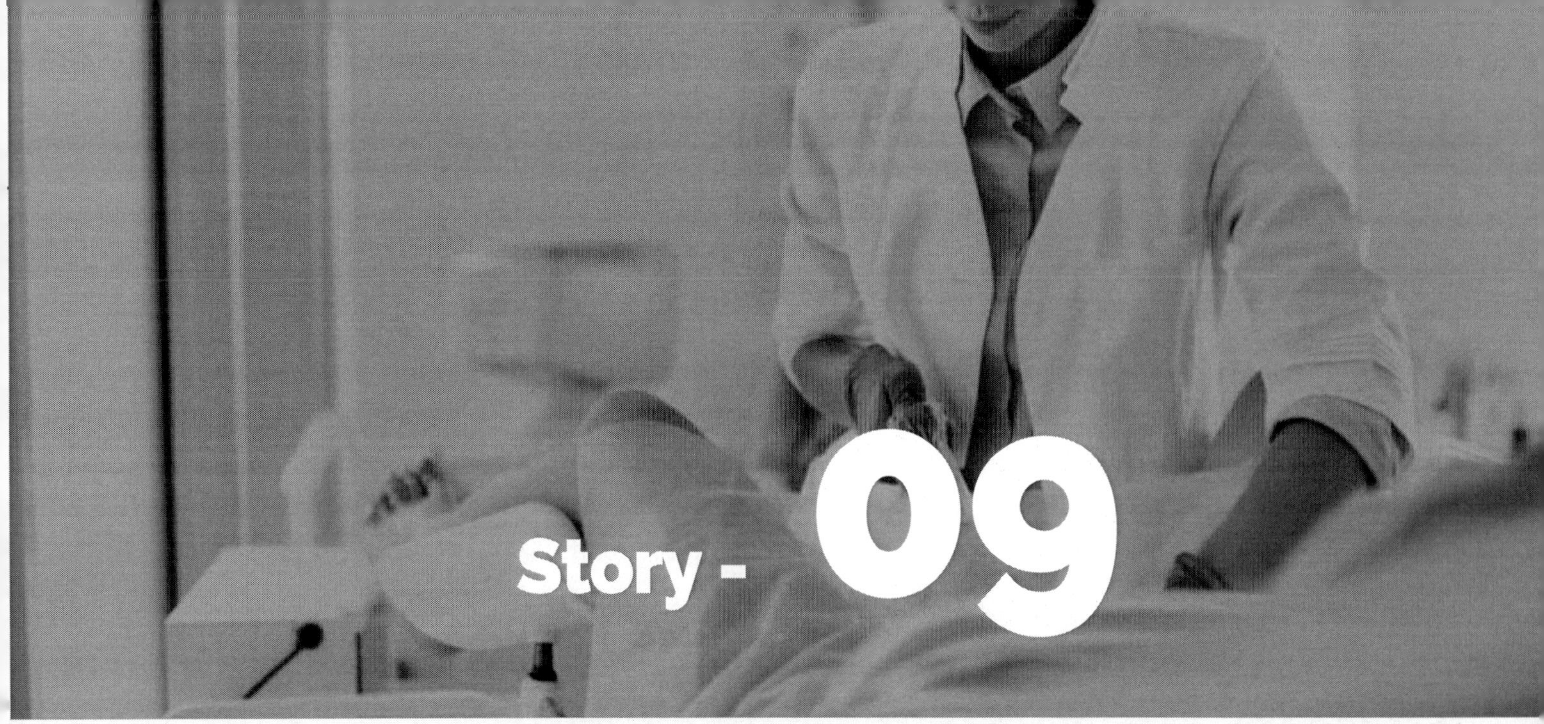

Unpredictable Gynecological Exam

Performing gynecological exams is one of the most essential preventative exams that I know of, indeed, right up there with breast exams and colonoscopies. A gynecological exam is performed every year or every few years, depending on the latest information, risk factors, need, and much more. Some women feel not a single ounce of anxiety about the exam, while others would prefer to have all their teeth pulled out. As you would largely expect, many of these exams could be described as unpredictable gynecological exams.

Some patients prefer women providers for the exam, while others prefer men. And even others don't have a preference at all. I've heard that some women providers can be too rough and some men to delicate. Regardless, a gynecological exam is very private, and for some people, it can be overwhelming. Finding the right person, if possible, is essential for some women.

There are many reasons why someone might be nervous about this type of exam. Our office tries to reassure each and every patient. I've had long discussions to try to alleviate some of the concerns. I've been performing gynecological exams for years and have many stories. Sometimes previous trauma could be a reason. Many women don't like other men or women to see their private parts, and there are other possible reasons.

One individual, in particular, had a story that was quite funny and unexpected. The patient hadn't been to see me in a few years. She was always super nervous about this particular exam. She was so nice. She called our front office and set up an appointment. She arrived fifteen minutes early, sat in her car for twenty minutes, came up to our door, and walked back to her car. She finally stepped into our office thirty minutes late.

The nurses brought her back to the exam room, and she was fidgeting and avoiding eye contact the entire time. She remained polite but withdrawn. Inside the exam room, her blood pressure was elevated, and she was hyperventilating. She appeared uncomfortable and anxious.

After the screening portion of the assessment, my nurse asked her to get undressed, and she left the room. A few minutes later, I came in.

Mrs. Blankton was pacing back and forth, half undressed. She had a gown but still had on her jeans. She was talking with herself, sort of psyching herself up for the exam. I could hear her and smiled when I came in. When she saw me, her face turned bright red.

I told her to sit down and just talk to me. We went over her medications, her menstrual periods, her pregnancy history, and such. My goal was to calm her down. It worked, for the most part. She calmed down until it came time for the exam. Logically she understood that she needed the exam. Emotionally she wasn't so sure. Again, this is quite common.

She made excuses about smells, shaving, and much more. Again, very common. And in most cases, most providers don't worry about any of these issues and more. We try at all times to be as professional as possible. I called in my nurse to assist. Mrs. Blankton undressed and quickly wrapped the gown around her legs and lay on the exam table.

My nurse got everything prepared, and I continued to talk and encourage Mrs. Blankton. I was standing next to her so she could see me. Finally, it was time for the exam. I sat on my stool, the necessary items in hand, and glanced up. Unable to control myself, I let out a loud laugh. It was my turn to be embarrassed.

Without stopping, I continued with the exam and finished. Mrs. Blankton shot up to get dressed; she was so red in the face.

I said, "Before you get dressed, can we talk?"

Mrs. Blankton, in a highly anxious voice, said, "Is everything alright?"

I said, "Yes, of course."

Mrs. Blankton asked, "Then why did you laugh?"

"Did you spray something before coming in?" I asked.

"Yes. I was so nervous about the smell that I grabbed my daughter's perfume. Is that why you laughed?"

"I see. Well, there's one problem, though. That was glitter spray make-up that you sprayed and not perfume. You were sparkling."

Mrs. Blankton was mortified. But in the end, after she cleaned herself up and got dressed, she laughed pretty well about it too. I've seen her several times since then, and she's had no problems with any further gynecological exams. I guess she made it through the "worst case scenario" and has been anxious free since then.

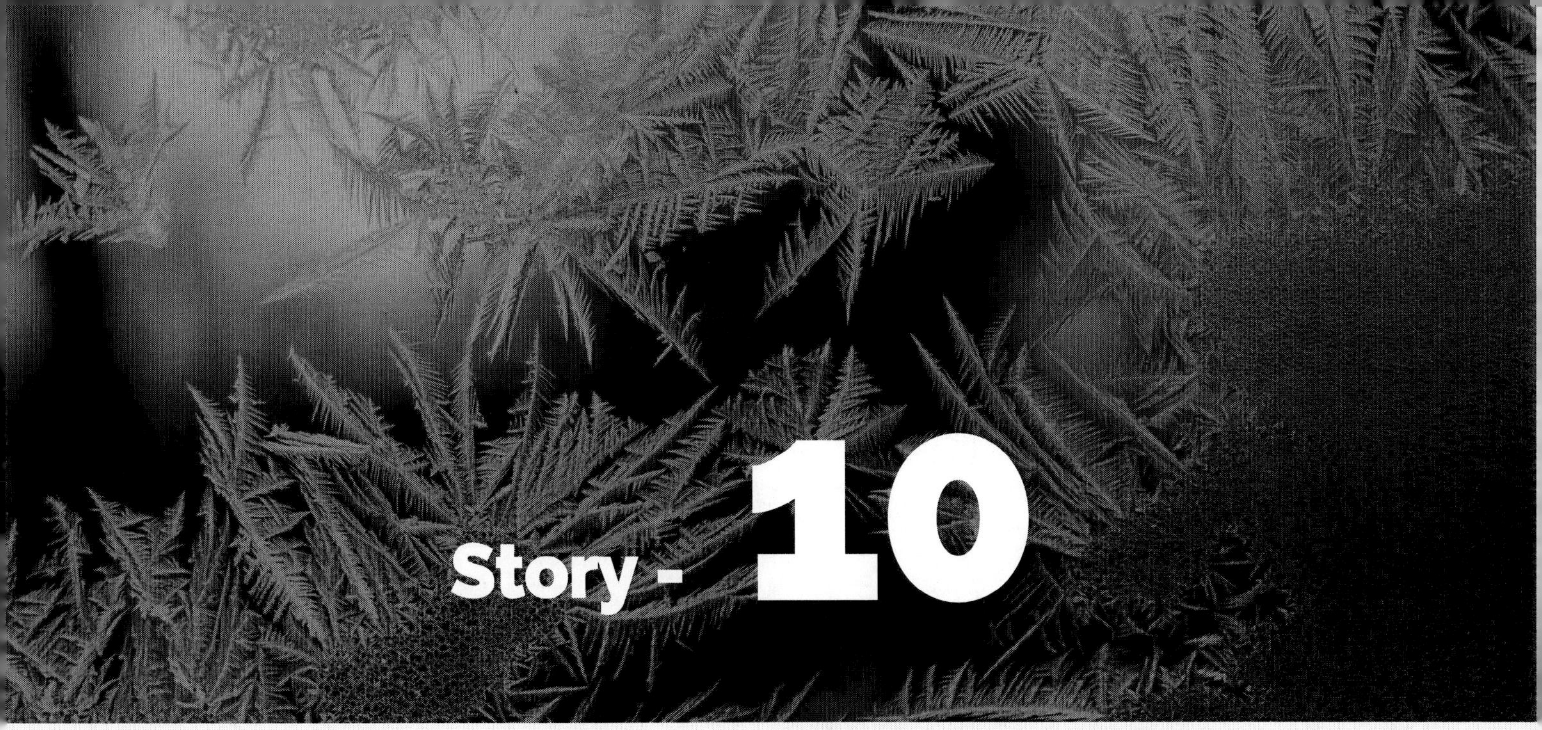

A Little Frostbite Doesn't Bother Me

A homeless patient named Beaver came into our free clinic to have an exam for the first time in six months. This was the name he gave when signing in. He was complaining that his toes needed to be looked at and that there was something wrong.

He explained that he'd been out in the middle of Wyoming when his car had broken down last winter. When he came into our clinic, it was the middle of June, and it was hotter than you can imagine. Continuing his story, Beaver said that he didn't have a cell phone at the time of his car's breakdown, and instead of waiting for someone to drive by and help, he began walking. It took him over an hour to walk the four miles to the gas station. Making matters worse, there were several inches of snow on the ground, and the temperature was below freezing.

At the gas station, he called his family, and they came and picked him up. Later that night, his toes started burning with pain. Over the next few days, he watched as the tips of his toes began to turn black. A week later, he went with some other friends and towed his car back to a garage to be worked on. In the end, he never went to the hospital or had anyone look at his toes.

As he finished the story, I had a sinking feeling of what I was going to find. This was not helped by the smell permeating the exam room. I feared Frostbite. I told him that the emergency room might be better able to help him. He explained that he didn't have the money.

He reported that his current symptoms were nausea, fever, and chills over the last week, but he felt lucky because the pain had resolved after the first few months. He was coming to our homeless clinic because of the fever and chills. He described plenty of numbness and tingling in both feet – but he reported that one foot was worse than the other.

When prompted, he quickly removed his shoes and socks. The site was pretty concerning. Several of his toes were black. I asked him if the blackness had become worse over the last few weeks or months? He honestly replied that he didn't know. He hadn't had a chance to clean his toes in months.

His right foot was the worst, and the first toe was most significantly affected, as it was entirely black. The second and third toes had a noticeable amount of color changes.

Frostbite is when the coldness of the air, ice, water, or whatever, causes damage to the tissue affected. Blood flow to that area is greatly affected. Over time, depending on severity, some of the skin may have a return of blood flow and an improvement in the skin. That was definitely not the case for Beaver.

After six months, the likelihood of saving blackened skin was doubtful. I continued my exam of the entire foot. He had sensation in the foot, ankle, and most of the outside toes. When I touched the dead skin on the first digit, it moved slightly and was dry. There was absolutely no blood flow to parts of each toe.

I began explaining my concerns about a possible infection, death of the skin, and the need for removal of the skin and further examination like an X-ray, MRI, and blood work. There was someone that I knew who could help, and I went to make the phone call for an appointment. After consulting with another provider, it was decided that the patient would have a small surgery and evaluation of the skin, bone, and tissues. Returning to the patient, I explained the plan.

He was deeply troubled by his toes and had difficulty getting past the blackness of the skin and what it meant. And although he hadn't done anything for the last six months, he wanted to have surgery and a more specialized evaluation today. I explained that an appointment today was not possible, but that one was scheduled for tomorrow. I spent a decent amount of time explaining what was expected, and Beaver left the homeless clinic far happier than when he'd arrived.

My medical assistant printed him out the antibiotic prescription and pain medications, along with the directions to tomorrow's appointment. Before he left, she cleaned the site and bandaged it as best as possible.

The next day, early in the morning, Beaver marched back into the clinic with a smile on his face. My medical assistant quickly came and found me, and I hurried out to the front room to talk with him. He explained that he couldn't afford to go to the specialist. I tried explaining that the cost would be covered. He replied that he only trusted me to help him but that he'd "taken care of the situation himself". I had no idea what this meant.

Beaver was rushed back into an exam room while I finished up my current appointment. When I arrived at his room, he explained that after he left the clinic yesterday, he found some dental floss and began cutting off the dead tissue on his own. He twisted the dental floss back and forth. The smaller toes had been less of a problem. It took him an hour to cut off the skin from the big toe.

By removing his sock, he allowed me a better examination. All the black tissue was indeed gone. Because the skin had died long ago, the real problem was the open wound and his lack of cleaning of the area. Pointing to the top of the first digit, I showed him where the bone was sticking out of the great toe.

He wasn't worried in the slightest. I spent several minutes explaining that an infection of the bone was possible. He argued that if he hadn't had an infection by this point, he doubted one was going to happen. I reminded him of the nausea, fever, and chills that he'd had yesterday.

Beaver said, "They are a thing of the past."

Beaver slipped back on his socks and shoes and left the clinic office without another word, whistling the entire time happily. I'd never seen anything like it.

Made in United States
North Haven, CT
10 November 2026

22106115R00020